AF877967

Dedicated to our fellow humans who lost their lives to the Ebola Virus, and to the thousands who are battling this disease!

Let's not panic!
Instead beat this threat with knowledge and awareness!

Chief Medical Author

Dr. Harpreet Singh MD, FACP

CEO and Founder | Vital Checklist | iCrush
Chief Medical Author | Vital Checklist Workbook for USMLE Step 2 CS (iCrush) Series for Patient Experience
Medical Educator | Vital Checklist Workshop for USMLE Step 2 CS
Chief Editor | Vital Checklist Blog
Patient Educator | iCrush Weight Seminars & iCrush Disease Seminars
Medical Advisor and Speaker | Vital Checklist & iCrush
Chief Organizer | iCrush 5k -The Healthy, Wealthy and Wise 5k

Associate Medical Author

Dr. Ankur Sinha MD

Executive Editor | Vital Checklist Blog
Associate Medical Author | Vital Checklist
Medical Advisor and Speaker | iCrush
Assistant Author | Vital Checklist Workbook for USMLE Step 2 CS

Associate Author

Gagan Pal Singh Ahluwalia

COO-Vital Checklist | iCrush
Executive Editor | Vital Checklist Blog
Advisor and Speaker | Vital Checklist & iCrush
Associate Author | Vital Checklist Workbook for USMLE Step 2 CS & iCrush Series
Creative Director and Branding Manager | Vital Checklist & iCrush
Head of IT operations and Internet Strategy | Vital Checklist & iCrush

Contributing Authors

Dr. Himanshu Deshwal, MD

Contributing Author | iCrush Ebola
Assistant Illustrator | Vital Checklist Workbook for USMLE Step 2 CS

Reviewers

Lena Chizek

Program Coordinator | Vital Checklist & iCrush

Illustrators & Artists

Mukesh Dutt Pandey

Gurmeet Singh

Table of contents

Preface

We at www.iCrush.org are true to our mission statement *“**Don’t tell the patient “What” to do, but tell them “Why” to do it!**”* We are a patient education and patient empowerment organization that stresses on improving the overall quality interaction between caregivers and patients. Our goal is to “**flip the clinic**” by empowering the patients to ask the right questions. Our mission is “**patient education at the fingertips.**” Our vision is **“early to diagnose, early to treat makes the patient healthy wealthy and wise.”**

Ebola Virus infection has caused a global wave of panic. We have used easy to understand **layman language** in order to send the message across. We believe in **empowering** the people in making their own healthcare decisions and protecting themselves. In addition to this book, we have made a dedicated website in order to spread awareness about the disease. The website contains a **free patient education video** that is targeted at educating people about Ebola within **5 minutes**. (www.icrush.org/ebola)

A lot of research from **numerous credible resources** went into designing the book. We have gone through various research papers and the most current recommendations from the CDC have been incorporated into this book to make it as accurate and current as possible. Information about this virus changes everyday, this book is current as of the date of publication. We will try to incorporate developments in our subsequent editions.

Special mention goes to **Dr. Ankur Sinha MD,** a budding physician from the United Kingdom, who has helped me write this book. He worked with me to develop the mnemonics, produce the patient education video and make the website www.icrush.org/ebola. He has co-managed the entire Vital Checklist & (iCrush) team and was immersed 24X7 in this project. Thanks to him we were able to complete this book in mere five days. He is an excellent Doctor and I wish him good luck in all his future endeavors.

We would love to communicate with you. This book is our first attempt, and there might be some inadvertent errors. Please email me at drsingh@vitalchecklist.com. We would surely appreciate any feedback and will incorporate in the next edition.

Let’s (iCrush) Ebola!

Harpreet Singh MD FACP
Grand Rapids, MI

Disclaimer

Medicine is an ever-changing and ever evolving science. Clinical experiences and research broaden our knowledge and understanding of a subject on a daily basis. The authors and publishers of this work have checked the information material for accuracy from multiple sources, and believe that the knowledge is generally in accord with the standards that are acceptable at the time of publication. However, in view of the possibility of human error, and changes in medical science, neither the authors nor any other party involved in the publication of this book claim that all information contained in this book is accurate in all respects or complete. They disclaim all responsibility for any errors or omissions or from any results that were obtained from use of the information contained in this material. This material is for informational purposes only.

The content is not meant to be a substitute for professional medical advice, diagnosis or treatment. Always seek the advice of your physician or other qualified health provider with any questions you may have regarding a medical condition. Never disregard medical advice or delay in seeking it because of something you have read here.

We do not endorse or recommend any tests, physicians, products, procedures, opinions or any other information that may be available on the website. Reliance on any information provided by the Vital Checklist website, the (iCrush) website, (iCrush) patient education booklets, the Vital Checklist employees or others appearing on the website or visitors is solely at your own risk.

Sincerely,
Vital Checklist and iCrush Team.

Dr. Harpreet Singh, MD, FACP

Founder & CEO - Vital Checklist, iCrush

I used to stutter. I was bullied, made fun off, boxed around and teased because of my speech impediment until 10th grade. I used to make acronyms (mnemonics) to overcome this problem. I never knew that I would be starting an organization that would coach patients, medical students and caregivers using these mnemonics. I feel that God has a plan for connecting these dots, from not being able to speak, to becoming an educator and a doctor!

I am blessed with an amazing brother-Dr. H. Paul Singh, who helped start my journey in America. I landed on American soil with 54 dollars, and he supported me through all the tough times.

In 2009, after my residency, I started a USMLE Step 2 Clinical Skills coaching institute and on witnessing the success of my medical students in their exams, I started using the same principles on my real-life patients. With God's Grace, I received numerous testimonials from my patients thus improving my Hospital Consumer Assessment of Health Care Providers and Systems (HCAHPS) score. On the teaching front, my students were passing the clinical skills test on the first attempt. On the patient front, I was getting numerous commendations.

Our Vital Checklist Workbook for USMLE Step 2 Clinical Skills for medical students is getting published, followed by Vital Checklist Workbook for Caregivers. We have used various theories to make the one **"Vital Checklist Theory of Patient Experience"** (ViCTOPE)

For the Patients, we want to provide a platform where they are connected and are healthy, wealthy and wise in making their own healthcare decisions. We want to **"flip the clinic"** by using various tangible Touch points- Communication Box, iCrush T-Shirts, iCrush5k, iCrush Weight Seminars, iCrush Disease Seminars and free patient education YouTube Videos. This platform is housed under www.icrush.org. Our vision is, **"Early to diagnose, early to treat, makes the patient healthy wealthy and wise."**

Through www.VitalChecklist.com and www.iCrush.org, we provide a communication platform for health caregivers and patients respectively. Trust develops through touching a patient with a soulful approach, in your head, from your heart and with your hands! Not just with technology. Technology is to assist, not to replace tangible human touch.

So Let's Love Communicating...

Dr. Ankur Sinha, MD

Associate Medical Author | Vital Checklist

Dr. Ankur Sinha is a young physician who recently graduated from Armed Forces Medical College, India. He went on to practice medicine in the United Kingdom soon after. He has always been enticed by the scope and potential modern medicine has, and plays an active role in developing new methodologies for improving the communication between doctors and their patients.

Dr. Sinha has been involved in the authorship and publication of many patient education books and articles. He believes that in addition to being immersed in clinical practice, a doctor can play several helpful roles in making their patient's lives better. He shares Dr. Singh's motto of bringing patient empowerment through patient education.

Dr. Sinha has exhaustively researched from various sources to make this book accurate and credible. His eye for detail and command on presenting complex content to the reader in an **'easy to read'** and **'hard to forget'** format have made this book truly unique.

Gagan Ahluwalia

COO & Creative Director - Vital Checklist, iCrush

Gagan Ahluwalia is the Creative Director and Chief Operations Officer at Vital Checklist and iCrush. As an entrepreneur and a highly seasoned tech, Gagan brings his penchant for perfection and experience to the team by means of active involvement in all creative ventures of our team.

His "non-medical" perspective blesses our structure of write-ups to be more layman understandable and helps reader absorb the content better. His insight keeps medical authors well connected with the readers shedding difficulties raised by unnecessary medical jargon. His aesthetic and creative genius aids in better demonstration of various complex topics in this book. He is a true asset to the development of this book by giving valuable inputs about making the book easy to understand.

Testimonial for Dr. Singh

This is a testimonial from Ms. Ashleigh Marie, one of Dr. Singh's patients.

"My relationship with Dr. Harpreet Singh started in May of 2013. I was one year away from graduating with my bachelor's degree in Psychology, I was a new homeowner with my husband of three years, and I was a young 23-year old mother of an infant daughter. I came to Dr. Singh after two years of unanswered questions from numerous medical caregivers. Since two years then, I had been feeling the sensation of numbness on my left leg. The numbness would come and go, but at times would last for weeks. A couple of times, the numbness was so severe that I visited the Emergency Room at our local hospital because I knew that something was wrong. Time after time, however, doctors checked me over and found nothing wrong. I was often sent home with muscle relaxants to deal with a "pinched nerve" that might be causing this numbness.

This same problem continued for two years until 2013 when I experienced another symptom that strengthened my belief that something was not right. That May, I started to fall down while walking. The falling would happen multiple times throughout the week. The falling was not due to me tripping over my own feet; the falls would rather feel as if my brain and legs were not communicating.

I remember being afraid. I remember not wanting to go to the Emergency Room ever again because of my previous experiences. How could I explain to someone that my legs and brain seemed to be disconnected?

I also remember looking through numerous Internet searches for a primary care physician in West Michigan who I could trust to actually listen to me. Through some divine intervention that I know had to be God, I found Dr. Singh. I had this tugging in my heart to call his office. I called and set up an appointment with him promptly.

When I first met Dr. Singh, he greeted me with a warm smile and a handshake. When he asked me to "explain" why I came in, I remember thinking *get ready for the muscle relaxers again*... but I was wrong. When telling him about the numbness in my left leg and the falls (I also had some double vision), I was ecstatic that someone finally was listening to me. He did not view me as someone who was just "complaining," he viewed me as a real person who needed help. He told me that we are going to be "very aggressive" in trying to figure out what was going on with me. He did elaborate clinical exam for 45 minutes. He ordered a series of blood tests, X-rays, physical therapy, and a MRI (magnetic resonance imaging) to rule out some possible diseases or conditions.

In the middle of July, after numerous negative results from all sorts of tests, Dr. Singh had the results back from the MRI. I remember Dr. Singh coming into the room with a somber expression-much different from the warm smiles he had greeted me with in the past. While he could not officially diagnose me, he told my mother and me that there was a good chance I had Multiple Sclerosis. (The diagnosis was confirmed shortly after, by a neurologist.)

continued...

Dr. Singh encouraged me to learn all that I could about Multiple Sclerosis as a disease as well as the treatments. He wanted me to learn so that I could then educate and help others. With the encouragement of Dr. Singh, I now share my journey with Multiple Sclerosis worldwide.

His acronym checklist for **"(iCrush) Multiple Sclerosis"** was worn proudly for "Team Ashleigh Marie" at the 2014 Walk for Multiple Sclerosis in Grand Rapids, Michigan. I am thankful for Dr. Singh and this learning tool that I can use to help educate the public about the disease, so many others and I are battling.

Dr. Singh and his acronym checklist for **"(iCrush) Ebola"** is something that is needed within a country of medical uncertainty. With this educational tool, the fear of Ebola, as well as numerous other diseases, can be silenced. His passion to educate his patients about the diseases they are battling is astounding. He believes that educating patients about their illnesses empowers them. Through educating patients (and the community) fear has no place to stand. Proverbs 27:17 says that, "iron sharpens iron." I believe that with the (iCrush) checklist for Ebola (and other diseases), Dr. Singh is doing just that; sharpening the minds of his patients so that they can educated not only themselves, but others.

My first appointment with Dr. Harpreet Singh lasted over an hour long, but I am so thankful that someone finally took the time to listen. His caring heart is something that he leaves as his legacy with his patients. That is something I will always remember and respect about Dr. Harpreet Singh."

- Ms. Ashleigh Marie

Introduction

The Ebola Virus has caused worldwide panic with the recent outbreak. Nevertheless, this virus can be contained if addressed with necessary caution.

Ebola is a non-segmented virus that belongs to the Filoviridiae family, which means 'thread-like' in Latin. The main genetic material in this virus is RNA, and its replication is the mode with which Ebola reproduces and multiplies in number.

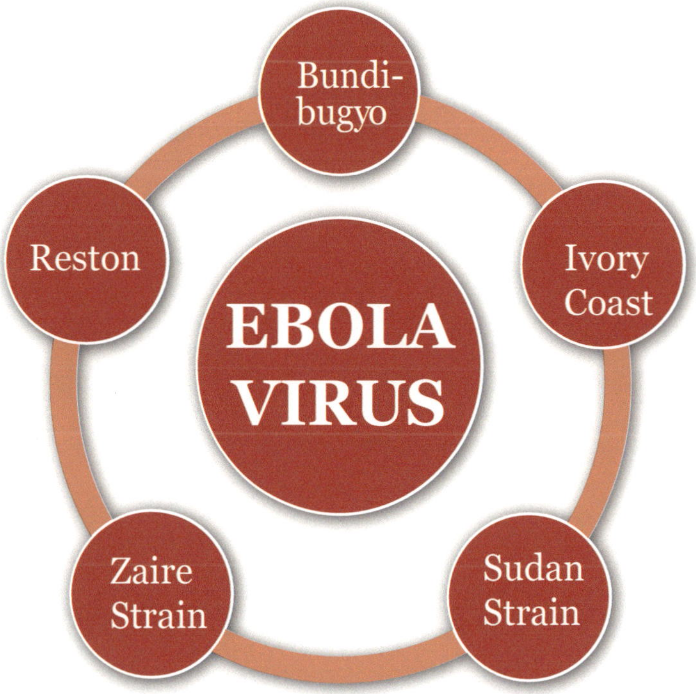

Ebola was first recognized in 1967. This virus has produced several epidemics every few years, but most of them have been isolated and limited to the African continent. The very first case of the Ebola Virus happened when infected monkeys were imported to Germany, and the kidneys were removed from these animals to develop the Polio vaccine.[1]

Five strains of the Ebola Virus have been identified so far. These strains of the virus have been named based on the geographical region that they were isolated from, and differ mainly in their amount of virulence, or in simpler words, their power of causing disease, and the disease outcome.[2]

Only four out of these five virus strains have posed a threat to humans.[3] The fifth strain, or the Reston variety, has never caused disease in humans. The present epidemic has been reported as the worst ever epidemic of Ebola, and started in the West African country of Guinea.[4]

How does the Virus Enter the Body?

This virus is constantly on the lookout for a weak spot on the body.[5] It lives in high concentrations in the body secretions of the affected individual, and waits to come in contact with another individual. [6]

The virus can enter the body if there is a weakness in the body's protective layers. This means that exposed mucous membranes and breaks in the skin act as entry points for this disease.

As of today it is understood that this disease does not spread through Airborne Infection.[1] This means the virus cannot spread through speaking or coughing. There is speculation about this, but no strong evidence to state that it spreads through the air. There has to be close contact with the Body Fluids.

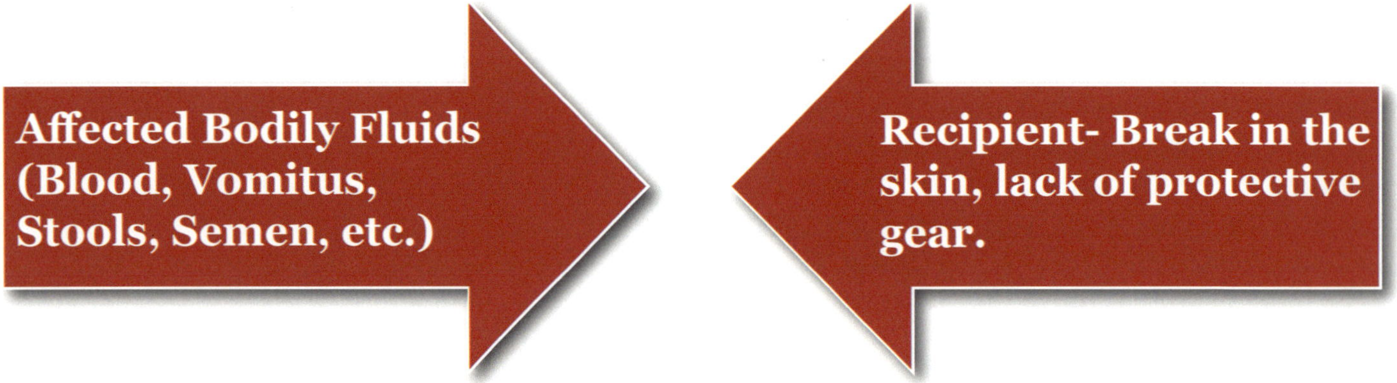

How does the Virus Work?

The Ebola Virus is very smart; when it affects the body, it targets the "guardian angels" of the body![9] These are known by the name of 'Macrophages', and their sole function in the body is protection from infection.[10,11]

Although the pathogenesis of this virus is not entirely known because it is difficult to do research under conditions of an outbreak, there is some data from laboratory studies on mice, rats and other animals in addition to what has been observed.

The macrophages, or the scavenger cells, are either fixed onto a structure or roaming around the body looking for germs to be killed. They are very similar to "cop cars" on patrol. When these cells come in contact with the virus, the result is catastrophic. The virus invades these cells and starts reproducing frantically.[12]

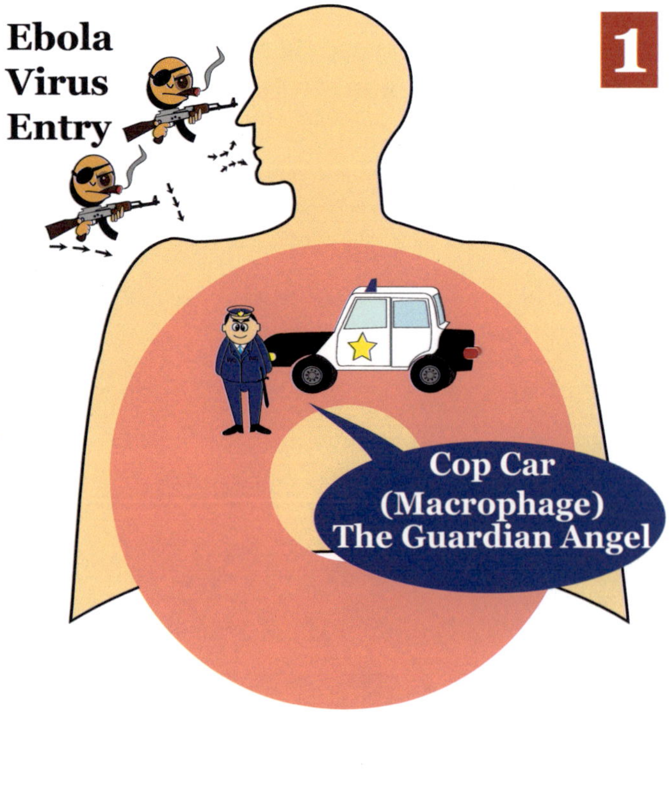

These viruses 'hijack' the macrophage cop car and take full control of it.
Eventually the number of the viruses increases to such an extent that the cop car bursts open and releases a huge load of virus particles. These virus particles are then picked up by other cop car macrophages, and the cycle continues.[13]

2

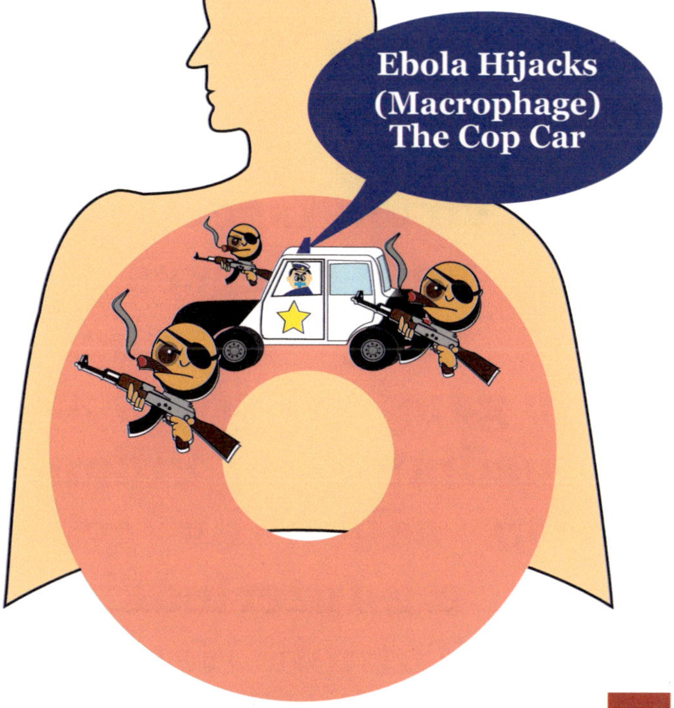

3

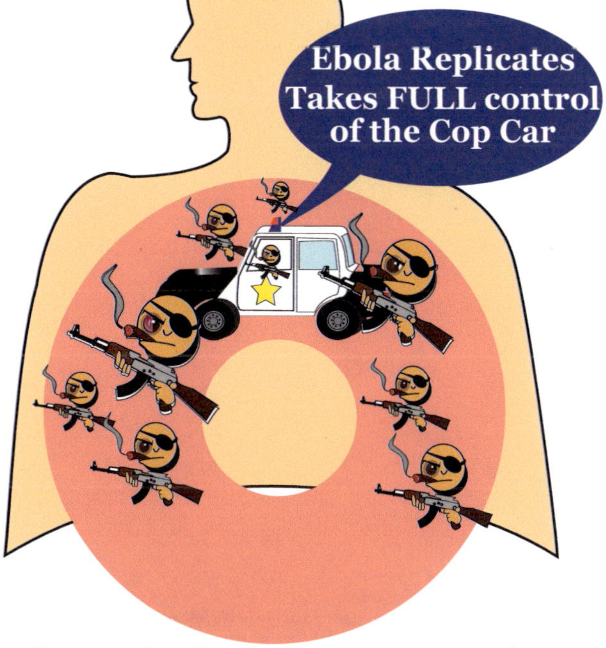

It replicates in the Cop Car (macrophage) taking control of it and becoming the commander in chief

4

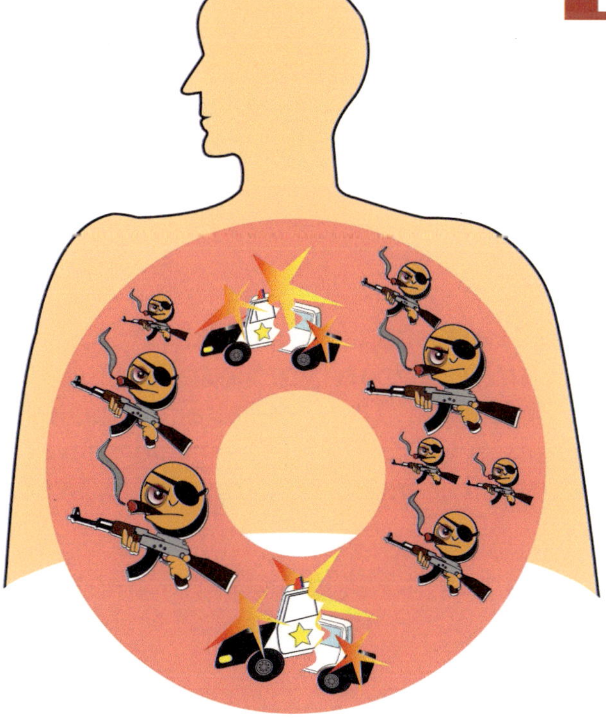

Virus invades the cell.

Virus replicates franticaly.

The cell eventually bursts open.

More cells are infected.

The Lymphatic System works like a drainage system in a house. Arteries provide nutrition and oxygen to tissues, and veins bring the blood back to the heart, meanwhile some fluid overflows. These Lymphatic vessels brings back overflow of fluid from the tissues. It has special nodes for specific regions that act as filters for the flow of fluid. These nodes have cells from the immune system of the body; the virus infects them as well. Eventually the body's defense mechanism is severely affected and it loses the ability to fight diseases.[14,15]

Now that the virus has replicated, it goes to the prison to free its gang members. These gang members are actually chemokines and cytokines (markers showing inflammation), and are responsible for causing the severe features of the disease.

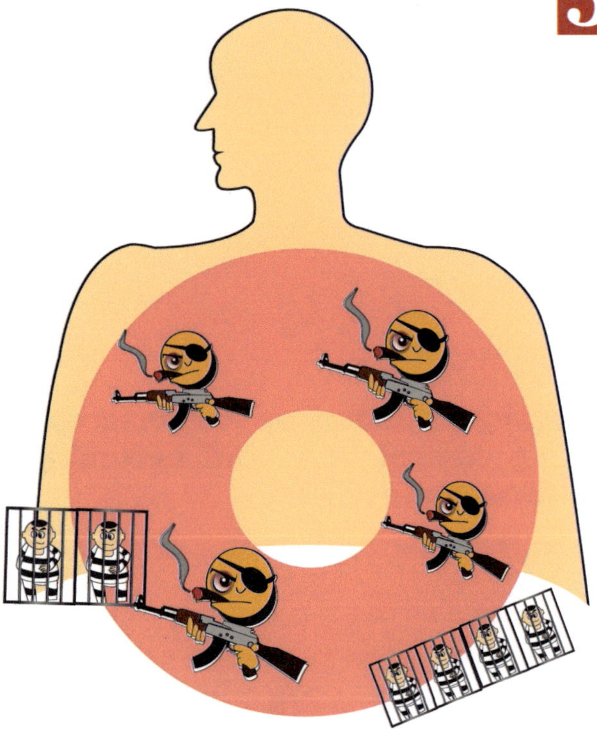

5 Ebola virus targets the prison and releases the other gang members. These gang members are the mediators of inflammation called as cytokines. e.g-Interleukin-6 (IL-6), Tumor Necrosis Factor-alpha (TNF-a) and Macrophage Chemotactic Protein-1 (MCP-1) and Nitrous Oxide (NO)

In reality, the virus causes damage to tissues, which leads to circulation of certain "distress signals" or gang members that the damaged tissue releases. These "distress signals" are basically cytokines and chemokines, namely TNF- Alpha, IL-6 and MCP-1 and Nitric oxide. These chemical mediators (gang members) are responsible for causing the severe symptoms of the disease. This includes fever, malaise, and dilation of the small blood vessels of the body, as well as increased permeability. In simpler words, fluid leaks into the tissues from the vessels.[16, 10.]

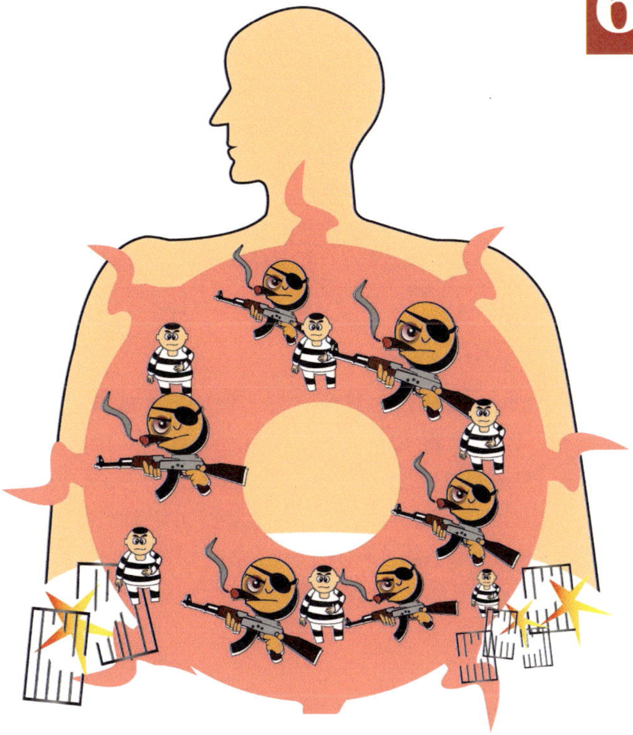

6

Together with the Ebola virus the gang members (cytokines) cause havoc and destroying the body machinery which causes leakage and hemorrhage from the blood vessels.

- Bleeding
- Shock (low BP)

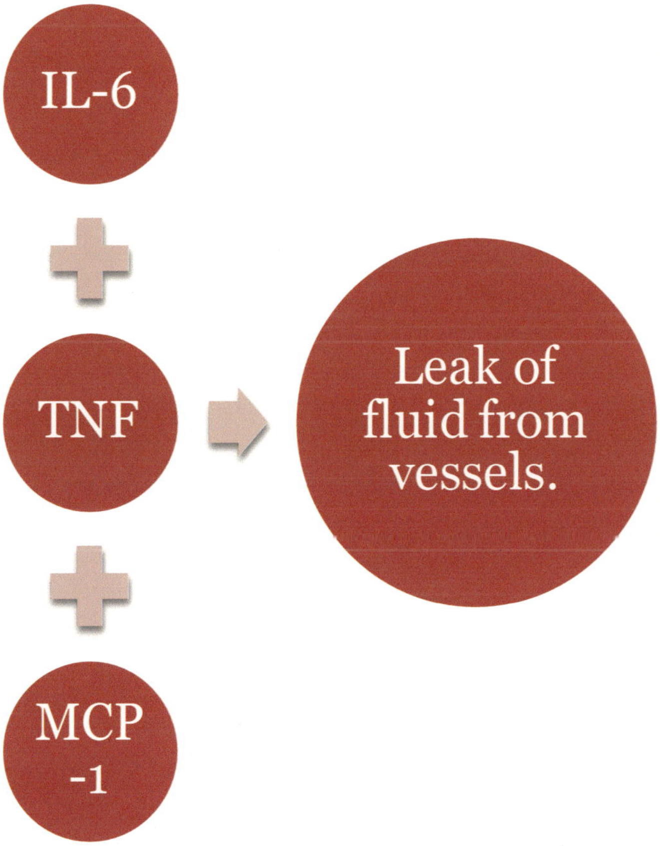

There is a significant disorder of the blood clotting system; this is because of the expression of a lethal feature of the virus.

Imagine an injury that has damaged the surface of a blood vessel. This event can be compared to a catastrophe that requires the platelets, who we call the “SWAT team” as well as the fibrin (fire brigade) or clotting factors, to come and help. Under normal circumstances, the SWAT team or the platelets, arrive within seconds and form a protective cover at the injury site. This is called the platelet plug. The fire brigade (fibrin), or the coagulation factors, follow and form a stable clot there. This clot is very important in protecting the body from bleeding out.

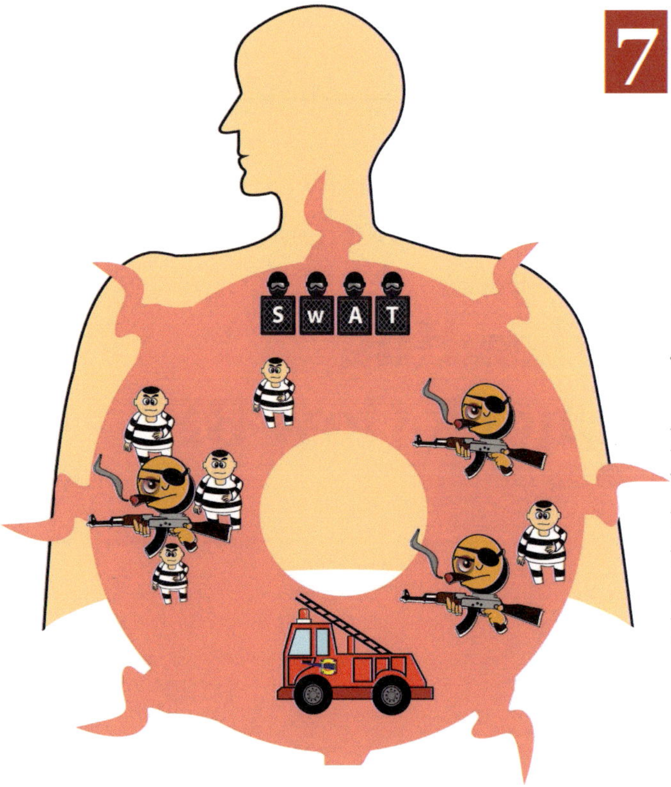

7

S.W.A.T Team (Platelets) reach the leakage site forming the first barrier to stop bleeding (platelet plug).

Meanwhile, S.W.A.T Team also calls the fire brigade (Fibrin) to stabilise the plug at the leakage site

Now this virus attacks this mechanism in two ways: the SWAT team is killed by the virus (Thrombocytopenia- low platelet count), and the fire brigade trucks collide with each other before reaching the site. (Formation of D-dimers or clumps of fibrin leading to depletion of all clotting factors.)[17, 18]

8

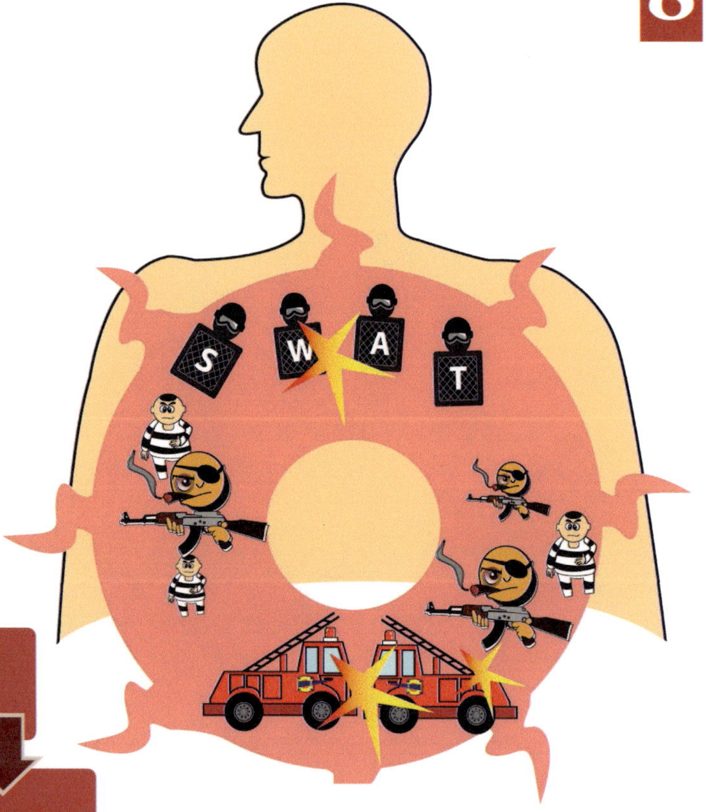

Ebola virus does not let the fire brigade (Fibrin) reach the site where S.W.A.T Team (Platelets) have formed the plug, breaking them down and colliding them with each other, forming fibrin degradation products (D-dimer)

This basically means that the body is unable to clot its blood when the need arises, and bleeds out.

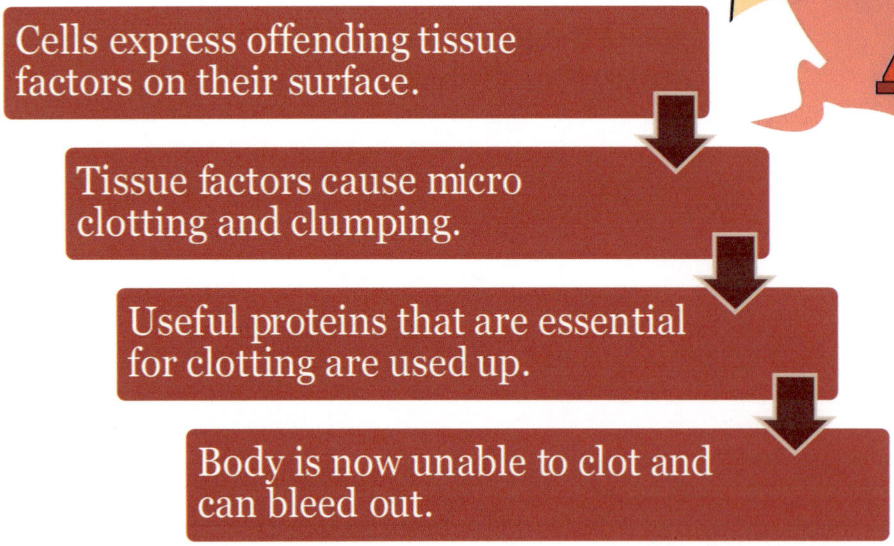

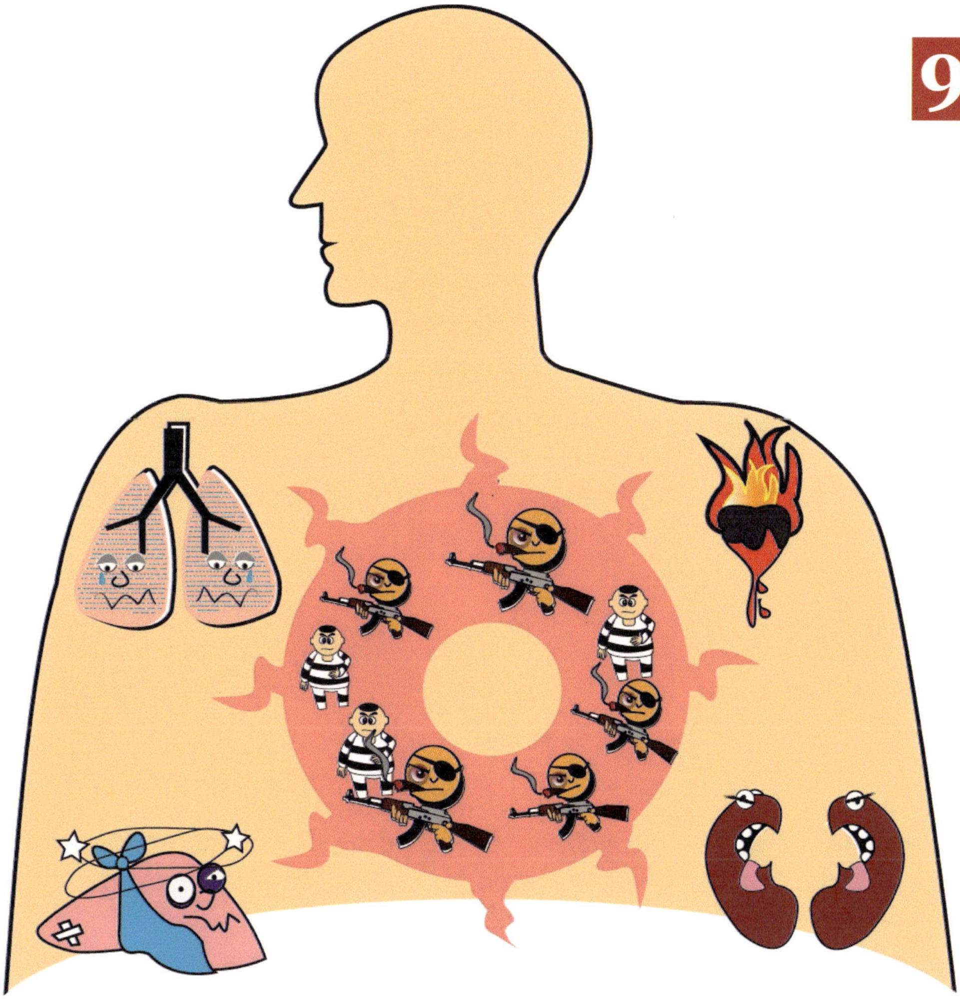

S.W.A.T Team (Platelets) fails to control state of shock (low blood pressure), decreased perfusion/blood supply to important organs, shutting them down.

- **Cerebral Edema**
- **Myocarditis**
- **Pulmonary Edema**
- **Renal Failure**
- **Liver Failure**
- **Disseminated Intravascular Coagulation (DIC)**

How can a person be exposed to Ebola?

The exposure to the Ebola Virus can be classified as primary or secondary exposure. The idea is that the virus can be transmitted by directly coming in contact with the affected animals in a territory known to have reservoirs of Ebola, or it can be transmitted from a person who has been infected by Ebola.[19, 20]

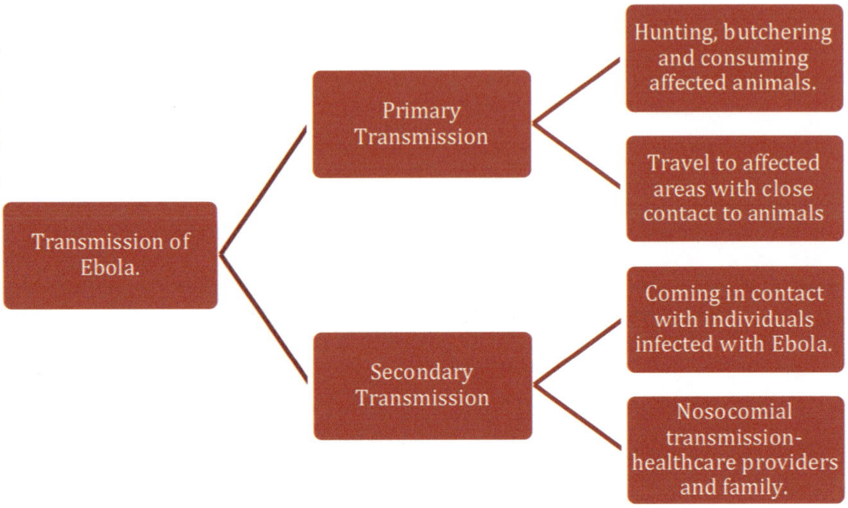

Who is at risk?

There is a huge amount of panic amongst people regarding the possibility of contracting this disease, and it is but natural to be worried. However, this disease is limited to a group of the population that is coming in close contact with infected individuals.[21,22]

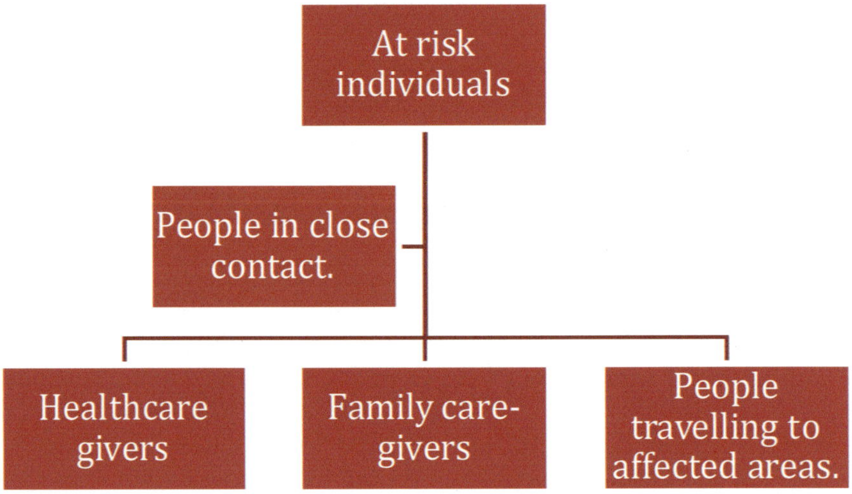

Family members may come in contact with the virus-rich bodily fluids while taking care of an individual. Special mention should be given to the ritual washing of the corpse that is undertaken in various cultures in preparation for the funeral, as the virus accumulates in the skin and sweat glands, and can be transmitted on scrubbing.

Healthcare givers can contract the disease in a similar fashion while caring for individuals. It is absolutely essential to use 100% barrier protection while taking care of the people that have been diagnosed or are suspected of having Ebola.[23,24,25]

Many cases of the disease results from the fact that the symptoms do not show themselves immediately following exposure, and the healthcare givers might be unaware of the risk. This is why the importance of universal precautions has to be stressed and regularly evaluated for efficiency.

What are the symptoms?

"(iCrush)Ebola" is an innovative *Vital Checklist* that is easy to remember and encompasses the common symptoms and presentation of Ebola. This Vital Checklist should be considered as a guide alone, and is not meant to replace a Doctor's Consultation. It is meant to help one understand the general presentation of the disease, and take necessary action sooner.[26,27,28]

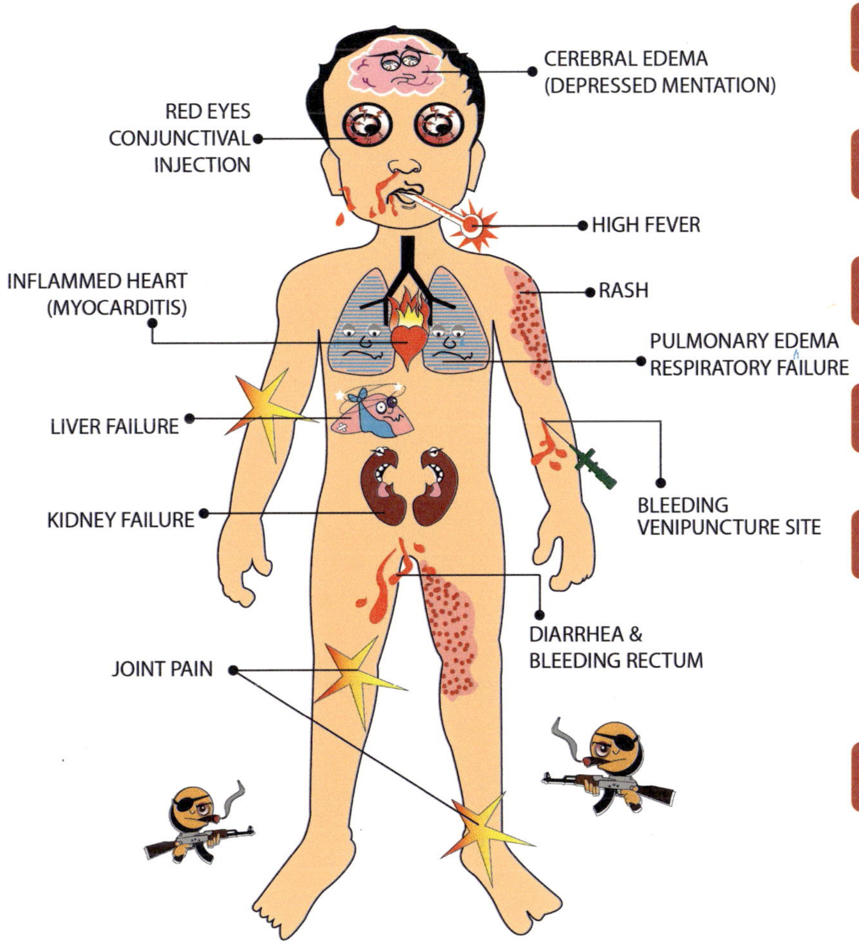

I- Initial Presentation

- Fever, weakness, cough and chills.

C- Conjunctival Injection

- Red eyes and redness of palate.

R- Rash

- Over arms, legs, trunk and face.

U- Urinary Proteins

- Early sign of kidney failure.

S- Stool, Seizure, Shock.

- Loose Stools with abdominal pain and vomiting.
- Seizure with nausea and headache.
- Shock with low blood pressure.

H- Hemorrhage

- Internal and external bleeding.

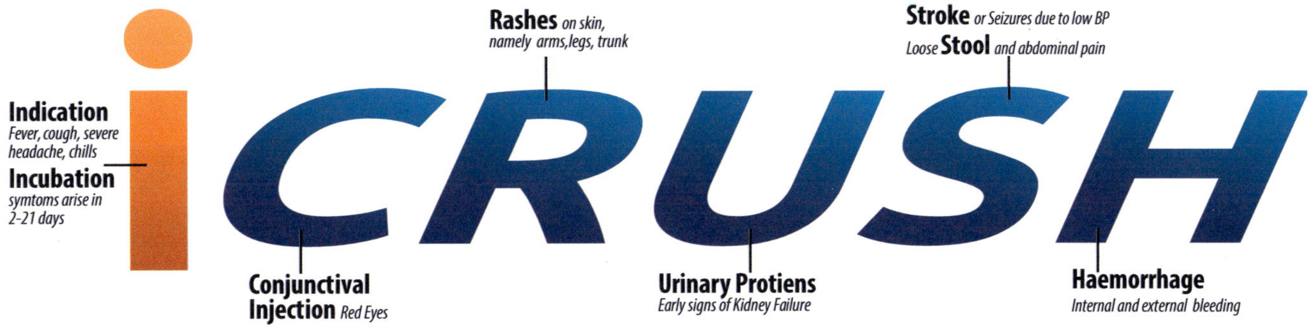

I- Initial Symptoms

This part of the checklist focuses on the initial presentation of the disease. Usually the affected individuals have an abrupt onset of their symptoms a few days after exposure. This initial symptom-free period is called the incubation period, and varies between 2 and 21 days. [29, 30]

The most common initial symptoms are non-specific flu like symptoms, like fever, chills, and general malaise. The patient could have muscle aches, nausea and cough without sputum.

C- Conjunctival Injection and Red Palates

This is also an early, and frequently occurring symptom. Paying attention to this symptom can help a layman pick up the symptoms of disease quicker and seek help in time. There is some involvement of the soft palate and parts of the hard palate as well; i.e. the roof of the mouth may appear red and swollen.

R- Rash

This symptom occurs slightly later during the disease. It has been reported to present at day 4-5 of the disease, when the other symptoms have made the disease apparent.
This rash is more evident in fair skinned individuals and most commonly affects the trunk, although it can involve almost all the body, and can desquamate or slough off.

U- Urine Proteins

This is actually a laboratory finding, but the availability of urine dipsticks in the household make it easy to test. This is also a late manifestation of the disease, and is usually a sign of the kidneys starting to get affected. Eventually the disease can progress to failure of the kidneys.

S- Shock, Seizure and Stools

These are serious and late symptoms. Five to seven days into the disease, the patient starts having loose stools accompanied with nausea, vomiting and severe abdominal pain.

Seizures and headache with confusion are late complications that show that the patient has a condition called cerebral edema, this means that the brain is swelling due to the disease process.

Shock is one of the latest and most profound complications of the disease. The term shock refers to the condition where the body is unable to supply enough blood to the organs in order to reach the oxygen and nutrition demands. This leads to severe injury to the vital organs like the brain, kidneys, and liver.
The main reason for shock is severely low blood pressure because of dilation of blood vessels, and a significant amount of blood loss due to ineffective clotting.

H- Hemorrhage

The virus causes the formation of a protein on the surface of affected cells, leading to the faulty activation of the coagulation process. This causes the useful proteins to get used up, and the body loses its ability to form clots.
This is also one of the late complications of the disease, and is manifested as bleeding through sites of venipuncture, petechiae, bruises and oozing from the mucosal surfaces.

What are the tests that can be done to detect Ebola?

According to the latest guidelines issued by the Center for Disease Control (CDC), the following tests are done to detect Ebola Virus. We categorize them as either early, or late, tests.[31, 32]

These tests are aimed at detecting the virus, or detecting the effects of the virus on the body. The ELISA tests are basically used to detect certain proteins formed by the virus. It works on the principle that if the sample includes the viral proteins, there will be a color change that can be detected by a machine.

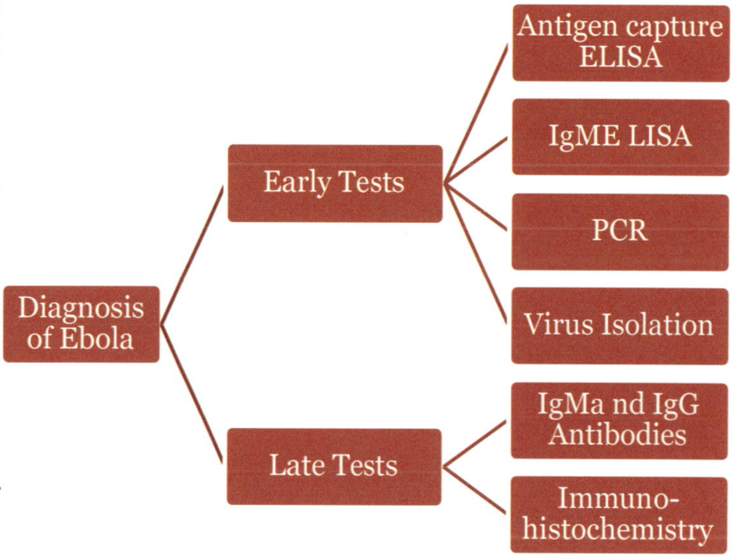

PCR works on the principle of catching hold of the genetic material of the virus and replicating it to an extent that it can be easily detected.

Virus isolation is difficult and mostly done after death to confirm the diagnosis.

Immunohistochemistry is done if the patient has not survived the disease, and a sample of tissue is taken and cured with the appropriate antibodies, and examined for a change.

Other Tests

Once the diagnosis of the disease has been made, some tests have to be done to assess the well being of the patient. These tests are:

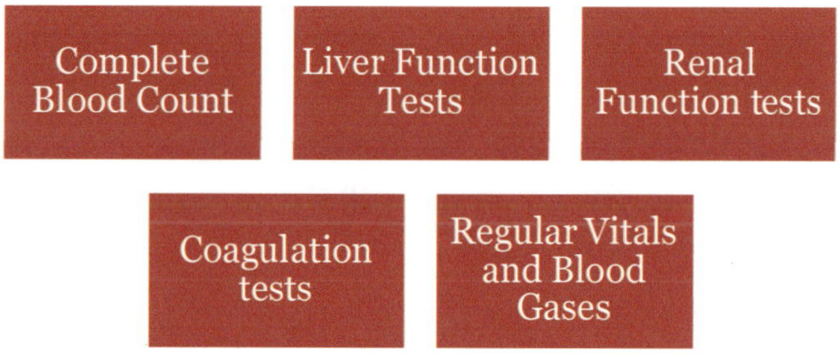

The complete blood count is done to detect the fall in the number of white blood cells that would be expected in Ebola Virus infection. It also serves the purpose of detecting a fall in the number of platelets; this is important to make sure that the clotting mechanism has not suffered.

The liver and the kidneys are severely affected in Ebola infection. These can be detected by keeping a strict watch on the levels of the liver enzymes.

Similarly, the renal function, or the kidney's well-being, is regularly tested to detect renal failure. Since the chances of the patient going into shock are high, it is mandatory to keep checking the vitals of the patient regularly as well.

What else could it be?

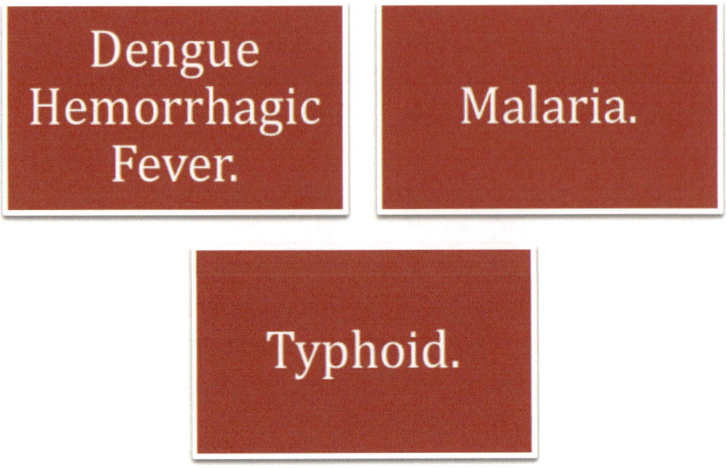

Making a diagnosis of Ebola can be difficult, and given the current state of panic, it is very easy to start thinking of Ebola at the first instance. It is very important that other causes of similar symptoms are ruled out, especially in the absence of **exposure** to a **sick individual** and **travel history**.

Dengue is a disease that can cause similar symptoms, and needs to be ruled out. It presents with high fever and severely decreased platelet count.

Malaria is a disease characterized by intermittent fever. There are associated chills, rigors, and splenomegaly is also a characteristic finding.

Typhoid is a disease that is characterized by a stepladder pattern continuous fever, this means that the fever rises gradually. There is associated abdominal pain, alteration of bowel and bladder habits and "rose spot" rash on the chest and trunk.

How do we manage Ebola?

Unfortunately, there are no definitive treatment options available for treating Ebola.[33] The management strategies are aimed at giving supportive therapy to patients, and helping them combat the disease. [34, 35]

The CDC has laid down guidelines for supportive therapy aimed at improving the outcome.[36]

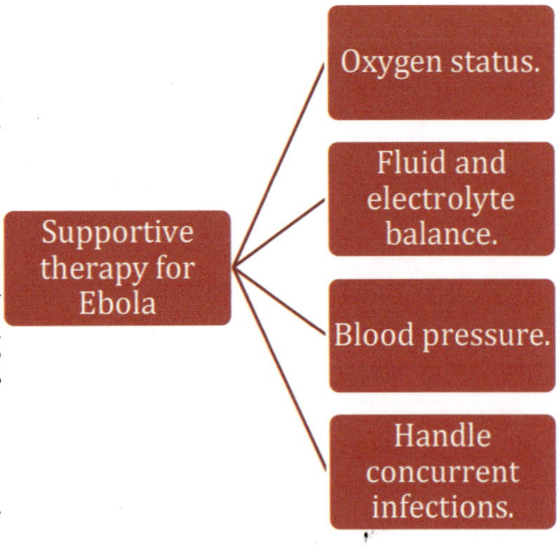

The first step towards giving good supportive care is **early intervention**. The oxygen status of the patient can be maintained by checking the oxygen saturation and administering oxygen by face mask or nasal cannula.

Intravenous (IV) access is a must to administer IV fluids. As mentioned above, affected individuals are at risk of having low blood pressure. IV access solves the dual purpose of maintaining the fluid and electrolyte balance, as well as giving vasopressor agents that can help in maintaining blood pressure. [37]

The body loses its power to fight infections and is prone to getting added infections on top of Ebola. This is called 'super infection.' Giving adequate antibiotics following blood cultures is a must to make sure that these infections are under check.

How do we prevent Ebola?

The best way to address the Ebola epidemic is to prevent transmission by strict universal precautions. According to the CDC, strict caution has to be practiced when dealing with cases of Ebola infection. [38, 39]

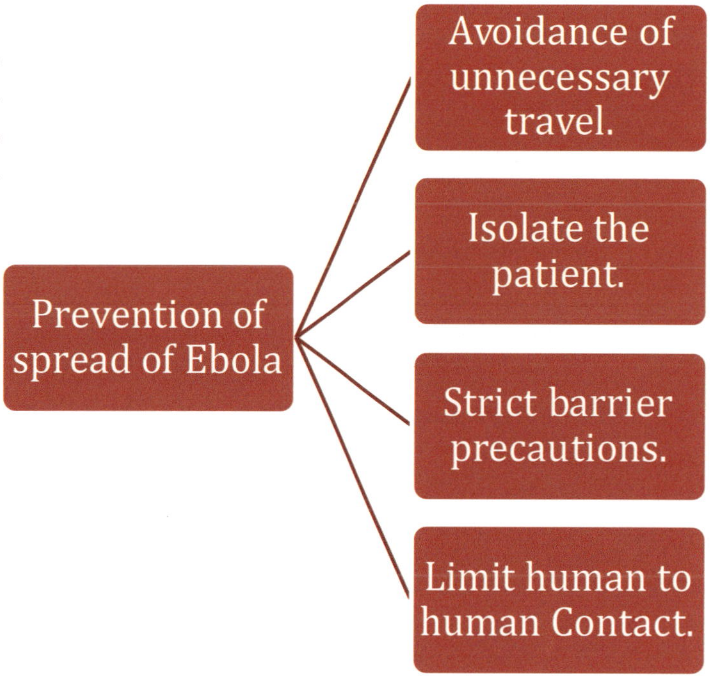

Avoid Unnecessary Travel

All travel to the endemic areas during the period of spread should be avoided. If travel is necessary, avoid visiting areas where patients of Ebola are being cared for, and treated. Avoid close contact with individuals who might have been exposed to the virus. If a person develops symptoms, especially within 21 days of coming in contact with an exposed individual or endemic area, please call and report to the CDC. Avoid using any public transportation and close contact with any family members while awaiting medical aid. [40, 41]

Isolate the Patients

The CDC has laid down specific guidelines for handling the care of patients in hospitals.[42]

- The patient should be placed in a private room with attached restroom facilities, and the door should remain closed at all times.
- Maintenance of strict records. Every person who has come in contact with the patient during the period of stay should be listed on a contacts list and monitored for signs of disease.
- In light of the current events, (when a healthcare giver was exposed to the disease and tested positive for the disease), personnel should be placed in the entrance to the patient's room. This would help make sure that barrier precautions are practiced efficiently.
- All medical equipment used for the patient should be discarded, or disinfected diligently if non-disposable.

Strict Barrier Precautions

Strict barrier precautions are achieved through the 'proper' use of Personal Protective Equipment (PPE).

- Proper application of PPE and removal should be practiced to avoid any contact whatsoever.[43]
- Limit the use of needles to the minimum, and disposal of sharp objects should be undertaken with the utmost care.
- All procedures that generate droplets of patient fluids should be avoided. Examples of these procedures include intubation and explorative surgeries. If necessary, make sure that these procedures are conducted with added precautions like disposable N-95 respirator, or higher protection respirators. All surfaces should be thoroughly cleaned after the procedure.

Limit Human-to-Human contact

This disease spreads through coming in contact with a person's bodily fluids. This can be easily avoided by limiting the chances of such an untoward event ever happening.

- Avoid entry of visitors into the patient's room- except health care givers wearing adequate PPE.
- All healthcare givers should be trained to employ universal precautions and proper hand hygiene. They should be monitored for symptoms and should report back immediately if sick.
- In the unfortunate event of demise of the affected individual, avoid funeral rituals or burial rituals that involve handling of the body, like bathing and scrubbing.
- Do not touch or handle items that have come in contact with the infected person's blood, vomitus or any other bodily fluid.

Is There a Vaccine for Ebola?

As of today, there are no FDA approved vaccines. There are some experimental vaccines, but they have not been adequately tested for use on humans. [44, 45]
Therefore, the strategy remains to avoid travel to endemic areas.

As of today, we don't have anything ready as a medicine, however with worldwide attention upon this virus, it is being extensively researched upon to mitigate this threat at the earliest!

We may soon develop a vaccine for this disease.

The Cause of Fever

Fever is a common finding with a number of diseases and people often wonder what causes it. We would like to explain the cause of fever using a simple metaphor of a household thermostat.

Imagine that the body is a big house and the hypothalamus (A small part of the brain responsible for a variety of maintenance functions of the body) is the thermostat. The thermostat or the hypothalamus has the responsibility of maintaining the temperature of the body.

Now the gang members (Mediators of inflammation that we talked about earlier, especially PG-E2)[46] target the hypothalamus and reset the temperature settings[47]. The body starts to think that it is supposed to maintain a higher temperature. This is done to make the environment in the body warm and cozy, this allows the viruses to grow.

The body like every house has some appliances to heat itself. This is much similar to the fireplace and the air conditioning in our houses.

The appliances are the muscles (Space Heaters), the Fat (The Fireplace) and the blood vessels (Air Conditioning). The muscles start contracting in a rhythmic fashion and generate heat, much similar to how the space heater generates heat for a room. This is why we have rigors.

The fat acts as the fireplace and a significant amount of fat is burnt to raise the temperature of the body to bring it up to the new set point. This is one of the reasons the core temperature of the body rises.

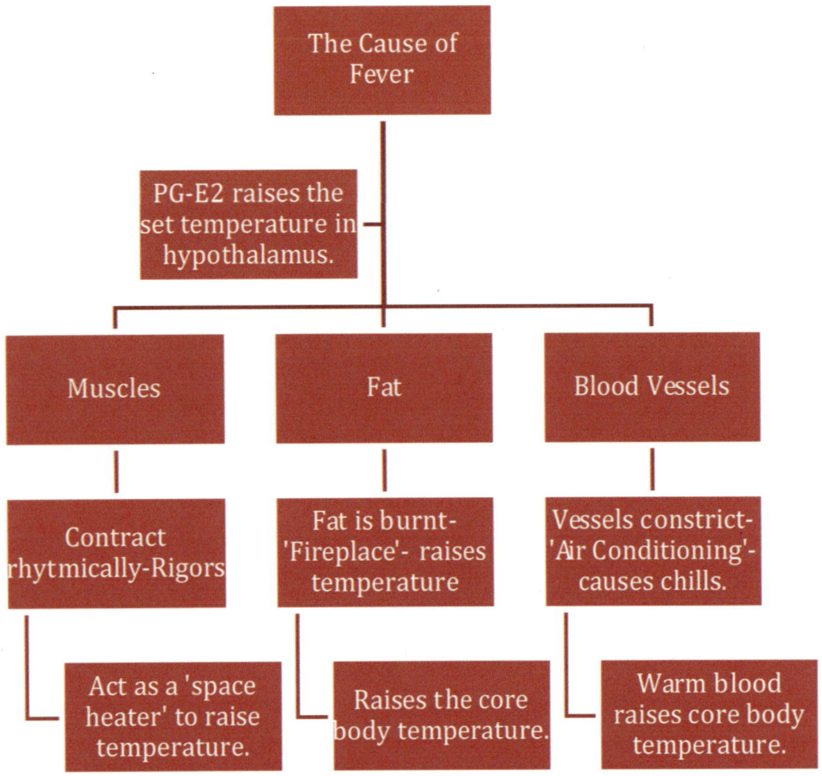

The blood vessels under normal circumstances carry warm blood to the limbs and skin to keep it warm and moist. Under the new circumstances the temperature set point has been raised. The blood vessels of the skin and periphery of the body contract, leading to pooling of warm blood within the internal organs. This has the effect of raising core body temperature as well as makes the extremities cold.

This is the main cause of chills.

Latest guidelines for application of PPE

The CDC is revising the guidelines for correct application and removal of PPE[48]. We cannot emphasize enough on the fact that the healthcare givers need proper and vigilant training in order to use PPE correctly.

The salient features of the revised guidelines include-

- Rigorous and repeated training of healthcare givers.
- Making sure that there is **no skin exposure** at all while caring for Ebola patients.
- All healthcare givers at all times are supervised by a trained monitor who watches them put on the PPE as well as taking it off.

The following mnemonic makes it easy to remember the correct application of personal protective equipment. *(General idea about the process of PPE usage, and in no means should be used as a replacement for proper training.)*

A- check your Appearance.
Usually the first step, signifies the need to stand in front of a mirror and better visualize all of the steps involved.

B- Boots and Buddy.
The next step is wearing waterproof boots that go upto mid calf level or used in conjunction with leg covers and asking a buddy (observer) to make sure that all processes are adequately done.

C- Cover all surfaces.
This step involves the application of 1st layer of gloves and a single use fluid resistant impermeable gown that extends to at least mid calf level.

D- Disposable N-95 mask.
The CDC recommends Disposable N95 respirators or powered air purifying respirators.

E- Eyes ears and nose.
CDC recommends single use full-face shield instead of goggles that used to get fogged and caused unnecessary hassle. This is followed by surgical hood that ensures complete coverage of the head and neck.

F- Full body Apron and Full body suit.
This step involves the application of second waterproof apron that comes to the level of the mid-calf at least; this is in order to cover the top of the boots from any spills.

G- Gloves and go to the hot zone.

The final step is to wear the outer layer of the gloves and enter the hot zone (Ebola affected) premises. These layers can make an individual extremely exhausted due to the heat and dehydration. It is recommended that the time within the hot zone should be limited to 1 hour.

ABCDEFG of Guidelines

A

- Check your **A**ppearance in the mirror.

B

- Wear your **B**oots.
- **B**uddy to observe you.

C

- **C**over all surfaces.
- I mpermeable gown and first layer of gloves.

D

- **D**isposable N95 respirator or a powered air purifying respirator.

E

- **E**yes **e**ars and nose-F ull face sheild instead of goggles
- Surgical hood to cover the head and neck.

F

- **F**ull body second layer of waterproof apron that covers the opening of boots.

G

- **G**loves- the outer layer.
- **G**o to the hot zone.

What if you fly? A-B-C-D℠

The CDC has advised people against travel into endemic areas, but if you must travel, please make sure that you follow these precautions. The basic idea is to make sure that your body does not come in contact with the viral particles.

Please note that it is highly unlikely that you would get infected with Ebola just by being in the same airplane as a person who has been infected. This is from the fact that Ebola does not transmit via the airway.[49]

It is not fully understood whether the transmission of Ebola is increased in the enclosed environment of airplanes.

This easy to remember acronym is called **"What if you Fly? - ABCD."** This is a guide to safe and sanitary practices while travelling.

W- Wash hands frequently.

The adequate method to wash hands using soap is as follows[50, 51]

Hand Sanitizer.

It is advisable to always carry a TSA approved alcohol based hand sanitizer on the airplane. The appropriate use of alcohol based sanitizers can help fight against many bacteria and some viruses like influenza.[52] This method of hand sanitization is quicker than hand washing[53] and does not need water, paper towels and access to a faucet. You must sanitize your hands after you have been seated.

Ill- Do not travel if you are ill.

If you feel that you have started developing symptoms of fever, please make sure that you do not use any form of public travel and inform your local medical authorities immediately.

F- Flu Vaccination prior to travel.

It is advisable to get vaccinated for Influenza[54] given the fact that Ebola virus can mimic the symptoms of influenza. If you are vaccinated against influenza, the chances of such a situation arising where the flu causes a scare is minimized[55].

Use Tissues-F L Y.

While travelling make sure that you have a handy pack of tissues, this will help in the safe and sanitary practice of turning off the faucet, handling the lavatory seat, and touching doorknobs to entrances of public restrooms.

F- Faucet.

Use a disposable towel to turn-off the faucet.

L- Lavatory Seat.

Use the tissue to handle the lavatory seat.

Y- Yikes! Doorknobs and handles are also dirty.

Use tissues to handle doorknobs and handles.

A- Airline Passengers- Watch out if sick.

As an informed passenger, you should look out for people who are sick or are showing signs of an illness.

B-Buy your own drink (BYOD)!

Never share a drink with anyone, no matter how close you are to that individual. You would be surprised to know how many germs another individual can transmit through just sharing a glass/straw that he has used.

C- Cover your Mouth!

This is one of the most basic hygiene practices that you should follow in order to avoid spreading germs. Ideally use a tissue to cover your mouth and nose while coughing and sneezing. Air and small mucous droplets travel at alarming speeds through our mouth and nose when we sneeze and the several layers of paper in a folded tissue is the bare minimum required to stop the spread of diseases. Again, We are just mentioning general disease control hygiene.

D- Discard the tissue immediately.

Discard used tissues immediately. The tissues can act as a storehouse of germs and should be thrown away as soon as used. The hands should then be sanitized using the hand held TSA approved sanitizers.

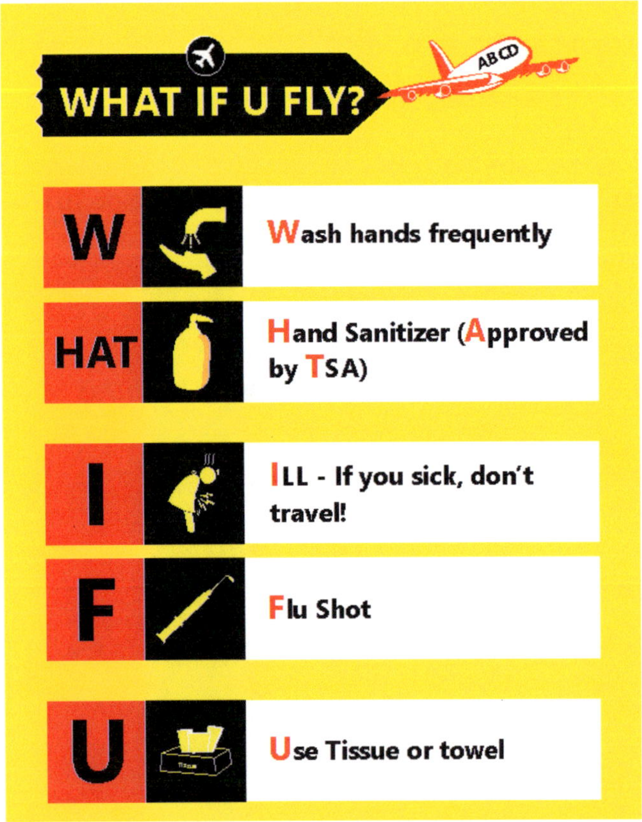

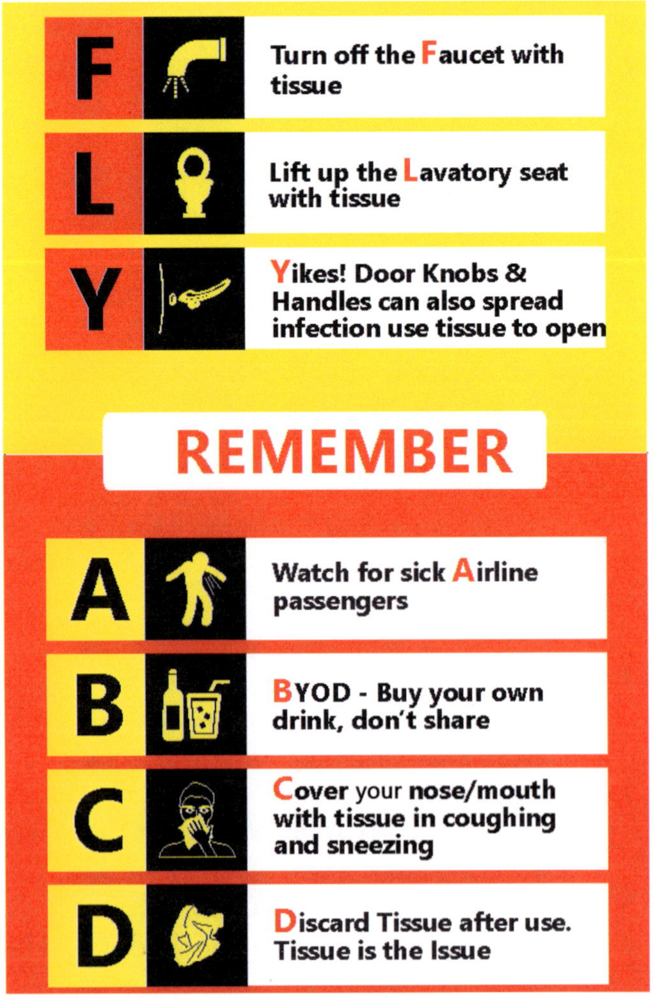

References (Endnotes)

1 Martini GA, Marburg agent disease: in man Trans R Soc Trop MedHyg.1969;63(3):295.

2 Bray M. Filoviridae. In: Clinical Virology, Richman DD, Whitley RJ, Hayden FG (Eds), ASM Press, Washington, DC 2002. p.875

3 Preliminary report: isolation of Ebola virus from monkeys imported to USA. Jahrling PB, Geisbert TW, Dalgard DW, Johnson ED, Ksiazek TG, Hall WC, Peters CJ, Lancet. 1990;335(8688):502

4 Ebola 2014 - New Challenges, New Global Response and Responsibility. Frieden TR, Damon I, Bell BP, Kenyon T, Nichol S. N Engl J Med. 2014 Aug;

5 Pathogenesis of filoviral haemorrhagic fevers. Mahanty S, Bray M. Lancet Infect Dis. 2004;4(8):487.

6 Centers for Disease Control and Prevention.Health adivosry network 367: CDC Ebola Response Update #3. http://emergency.cdc.gov/han/han00367.asp

7 http://www.cdc.gov/vhf/ebola/transmission/index.html?s_cid=cs_3923

8 http://www.cdc.gov/vhf/ebola/transmission/index.html?s_cid=cs_3923

9 Pathogenesis of Ebola hemorrhagic fever in cynomolgus macaques: evidence that dendritic cells are early and sustained targets of infection. Geisbert TW, Hensley LE, Larsen T, Young HA, Reed DS, Geisbert JB, Scott DP, Kagan E, Jahrling PB, Davis KJ. Am J Pathol. 2003;163(6):2347.

10 The Centers for Disease Control and Prevention. Ebola Virus Disease Information for Clinicians in U.S. Healthcare Settings, http://www.cdc.gov/vhf/ebola/hcp/clinician-information-us-healthcare-settings.html

11 Cutting edge: impairment of dendritic cells and adaptive immunity by Ebola and Lassa viruses. Mahanty S, Hutchinson K, Agarwal S, McRae M, Rollin PE, Pulendran B. J Immunol. 2003;170(6):2797.

12 Ebola virus: the role of macrophages and dendritic cells in the pathogenesis of Ebola hemorrhagic fever. Bray M, Geisbert TW. Int J Biochem Cell Biol. 2005;37(8):1560.

13 Pathogenesis of filoviral haemorrhagic fevers. Mahanty S, Bray M. Lancet Infect Dis. 2004;4(8):487

14 Defective humoral responses and extensive intravascular apoptosis are associated with fatal outcome in Ebola virus-infected patients. Baize S, Leroy EM, Georges-Courbot MC, Capron M, Lansoud-Soukate J, DebréP, Fisher-Hoch SP, McCormick JB, Georges AJ. Nat Med. 1999;5(4):423.

15 Functional CD8+ T cell responses in lethal Ebola virus infection. Bradfute SB, Warfield KL, Bavari S. J Immunol. 2008;180(6):4058.

16 Pathogenesis of filoviral haemorrhagic fevers. Mahanty S, Bray M. Lancet Infect Dis. 2004;4(8):487.

17 Pathogenesis of Ebola hemorrhagic fever in primate models: evidence that hemorrhage is not a direct effect of virus-induced cytolysis of endothelial cells. Geisbert TW, Young HA, Jahrling PB, Davis KJ, Larsen T, Kagan E, Hensley LE. Am J Pathol. 2003;163(6):2371.

18 Mechanisms underlying coagulation abnormalities in ebola hemorrhagic fever: overexpression of tissue factor in primate monocytes/macrophages is a key event. Geisbert TW, Young HA, Jahrling PB, Davis KJ, Kagan E, Hensley LE. J Infect Dis. 2003;188(11):1618.

19 Sensitivity to ultraviolet radiation of Lassa, vaccinia, and Ebola viruses dried on surfaces. Sagripanti JL, Lytle CD Arch Virol. 2011 Mar;156(3):489-94. Epub 2010 Nov 23.

20 Persistence in darkness of virulent alphaviruses, Ebola virus, and Lassa virus deposited on solid surfaces. Sagripanti JL, Rom AM, Holland LE. Arch Virol. 2010 Dec;155(12):2035-9. Epub 2010 Sep 15.

21 Centers for Disease Control and Prevention.Health adivosry network 367: CDC Ebola Response Update #3. http://emergency.cdc.gov/han/han00367.asp

22 The Centers for Disease Control and Prevention. Facts about bushmeat and Ebola. http://www.cdc.gov/vhf/ebola/pdf/bushmeat-and-ebola.pdf

23 World Health Organization. Unprecedented number of medical staff infected with Ebola. http://www.who.int/mediacentre/news/ebola/25-august-2014/en/#

24 Assessment of ebola virus disease, health care infrastructure, and preparedness - four counties, southeastern liberia, august 2014. Forrester JD, Pillai SK, Beer KD, Neatherlin J, Massaquoi M, Nyenswah TG, Montgomery JM, Cock KD. MMWR Morb Mortal Wkly Rep. 2014 Oct;63(40):891-3.

25 World Health Organization: Ebola response roadmap situation report: 15 October 2014 http://apps.who.int/iris/bitstream/10665/136508/1/roadmapsitrep15Oct2014.pdf?ua=1

26 Basic clinical and laboratory features of filoviral hemorrhagic fever. Kortepeter MG, Bausch DG, Bray M. J Infect Dis. 2011 Nov;204 Suppl 3:S810-6.

27 Piot P, Breman JG, Heymann DL, et al. Clinical aspects of Ebola virus infection in Yambuku area, Zaire, 1976. In: Ebola Virus Haemorrhagic Fever, Pattyn S (Ed), Elsevier/North-Holland, Amsterdam 1978. p.17.

28 The Centers for Disease Control and Prevention. Ebola Virus Disease Information for Clinicians in U.S. Healthcare Settings, http://www.cdc.gov/vhf/ebola/hcp/clinician-information-us-healthcare-settings.html

29 Ebola hemorrhagic fever in Kikwit, Democratic Republic of the Congo: clinical observations in 103 patients. Bwaka MA, Bonnet MJ, Calain P, Colebunders R, De Roo A, Guimard Y, Katwiki KR, Kibadi K, Kipasa MA, Kuvula KJ, Mapanda BB, Massamba M, Mupapa KD, Muyembe-Tamfum JJ, Ndaberey E, Peters CJ, Rollin PE, Van den Enden E, Van den Enden E. J Infect Dis. 1999;179 Suppl 1:S1.

30 The Centers for Disease Control and Prevention. Ebola Virus Disease Information for Clinicians in U.S. Healthcare Settings, http://www.cdc.gov/vhf/ebola/hcp/clinician-information-us-healthcare-settings.html

31 Basic clinical and laboratory features of filoviral hemorrhagic fever. Kortepeter MG, Bausch DG, Bray M. J Infect Dis. 2011 Nov;204 Suppl 3:S810-6.

32 The Centers for Disease Control and Prevention. Health Alert Network. Guidelines for evaluation of US patients suspected of having Ebola virus disease. http://www.bt.cdc.gov/han/han00364.asp

33 Infectious diseases. Ebola drugs still stuck in lab. Enserink M. Science. 2014 Jul;345(6195):364-5.

34 Ribner BS. Treating patients with Ebola virus infections in the US: lessons learned. Presented at IDWeek, October 8, 2014. Philadelphia PA

35 Caring for critically ill patients with ebola virus disease. Perspectives from west Africa. Fowler RA, Fletcher T, Fischer WA 2nd, Lamontagne F, Jacob S, Brett-Major D, Lawler JV, Jacquerioz FA, Houlihan C, O'Dempsey T, Ferri M, Adachi T, Lamah MC, Bah EI, Mayet T, Schieffelin J, McLellan SL, Senga M, Kato Y, Clement C, Mardel S, Vallenas Bejar De Villar RC, Shindo N, Bausch D. Am J Respir Crit Care Med. 2014 Oct;190(7):733-7.

36 The Centers for Disease Control and Prevention http://www.cdc.gov/vhf/ebola/treatment/

37 Ebola hemorrhagic fever and septic shock. Bray M, Mahanty S. J Infect Dis. 2003;188(11):1613.

38 Centers for Disease Control and Prevention. Infection prevention and control recommendations for hospitalized

patients with known or suspected Ebola hemorrhagic fever in U.S. hospitals. http://www.cdc.gov/vhf/ebola/hcp/infection-prevention-and-control-recommendations.html

39 World Health Organization. Interim Infection Prevention and Control Guidance for Care of Patients with Suspected or Confirmed Filovirus Haemorrhagic Fever in Health-Care Settings. http://www.who.int/csr/resources/who-ipc-guidance-ebolafinal-09082014.pdf with Focus on Ebola

40 World Health Organziation. Travel and transport risk assessment: Recommendations for public health authorities and transport sector. http://www.who.int/ith/updates/20140421/en/

41 The United States Centers for Disease Control and Prevention. Interim Guidance for Monitoring and Movement of Persons with Ebola Virus Disease Exposure. http://www.cdc.gov/vhf/ebola/hcp/monitoring-and-movement-of-persons-with-exposure.html

42 Centers for Disease Control and Prevention. Interim guidance for environmental infection control in hospitals for Ebola virus. http://www.cdc.gov/vhf/ebola/hcp/environmental-infection-control-in-hospitals.html

43 The Centers for Disease Control and Prevention. Fact sheet: CDC taking active steps related to hospital preparedness for Ebola treatment http://www.cdc.gov/media/releases/2014/fs1014-ebola-investigation-fact-sheet.pdf

44 Ebola Vaccination: If Not Now, When? Galvani AP, Ndeffo-Mbah ML, Wenzel N, Childs JE. Ann Intern Med. 2014 Aug;

45 Largest-Ever Outbreak of Ebola Virus Disease Thrusts Experimental Therapies, Vaccines Into Spotlight. Hampton T. JAMA. 2014;312(10):987.

46 Prostaglandin E2 and fever: a continuing debate. Coceani F, Bishai I, Lees J, Sirko S. Yale J Biol Med. 1986;59(2):169.

47 Prostaglandin E2 in the pathogenesis of fever. An update. Coceani F, Akarsu ES Ann N Y Acad Sci. 1998;856:76.

48 The Center for disease control and prevention- http://www.cdc.gov/media/releases/2014/fs1020-ebola-personal-protective-equipment.html

49 The Centre for Disease control and prevention- http://www.cdc.gov/media/releases/2014/faq1017-ebola-investigation-frequently-asked-questions.html

50 Healthcare Infection Control Practices Advisory Committee and the HICPAC/SHEA/APIC/IDSA Hand Hygiene Task Force. Centers for Disease Control and Prevention. Morbidity and Mortality Weekly Report 2002; 51(RR-16):1.

51 Evidence-based model for hand transmission during patient care and the role of improved practices. Pittet D, Allegranzi B, Sax H, Dharan S, Pessoa-Silva CL, Donaldson L, Boyce JM, WHO Global Patient Safety Challenge, World Alliance for Patient Safety. Lancet Infect Dis. 2006;6(10):641.

52 Reduction in nosocomial transmission of drug-resistant bacteria after introduction of an alcohol-based handrub. Gordin FM, Schultz ME, Huber RA, Gill JA. Infect Control Hosp Epidemiol. 2005;26(7):650.

53 No time for handwashing!? Handwashing versus alcoholic rub: can we afford 100% compliance? Voss A, Widmer AF. Infect Control Hosp Epidemiol. 1997;18(3):205.

54 CDC. Health information for international travel 2011-2012. DHHS, Atlanta, GA 2011.

55 Prevention and control of seasonal influenza with vaccines: recommendations of the Advisory Committee on Immunization Practices (ACIP), 2009. Fiore AE, Shay DK, Broder K, Iskander JK, Uyeki TM, Mootrey G, Bresee JS, Cox NJ, Centers for Disease Control and Prevention. MMWR Recomm Rep. 2009;58(RR-8):1.

Coming soon... More such Patient Education Booklets on

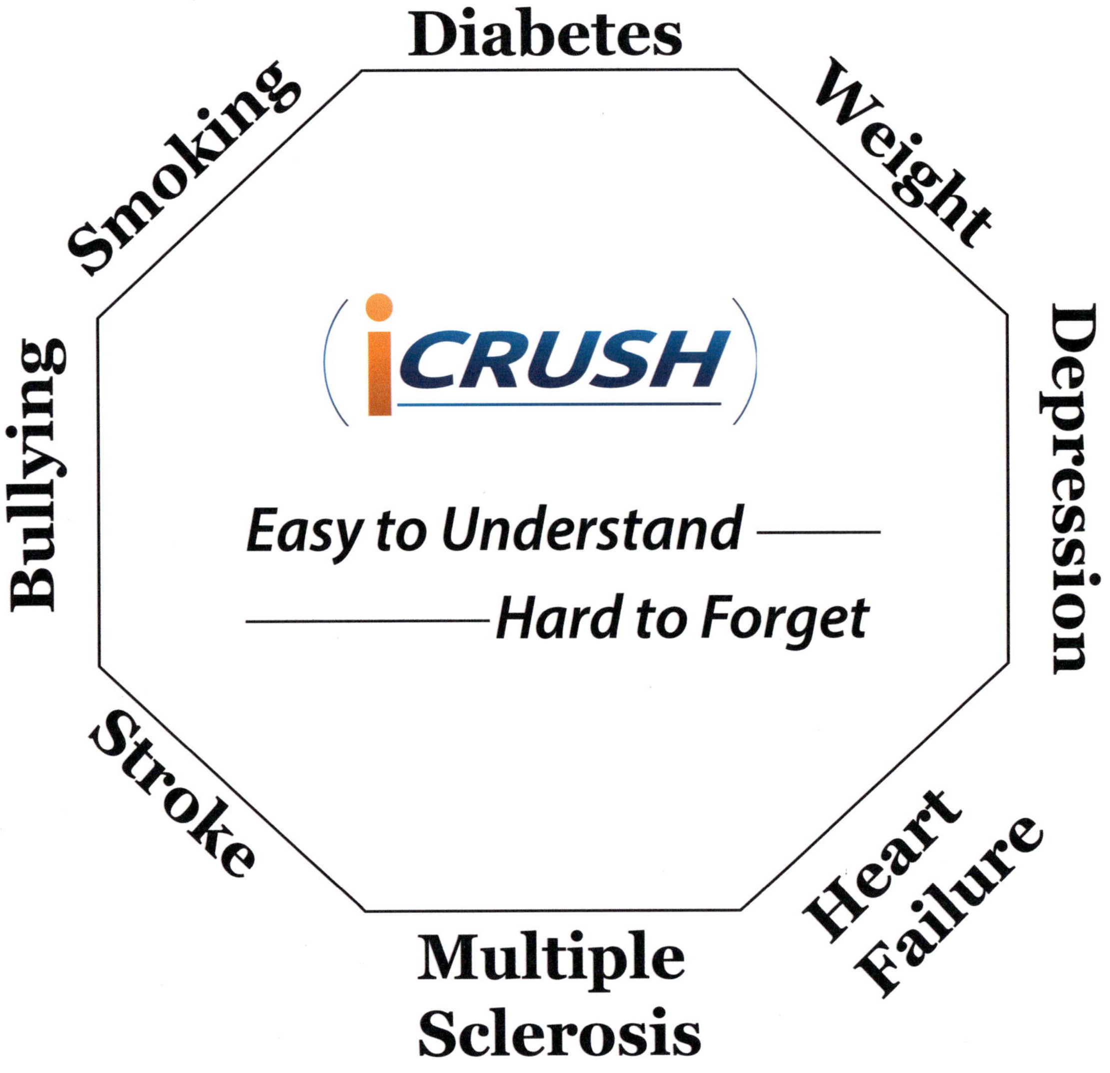

Log into www.iCrush.org to find next :

iCrush Walk/Run/5K

iCrush Weight seminar

iCrush Disease seminar